I0490525

Arthritis is a common condition that affects millions of people worldwide, causing pain, inflammation, and stiffness in the joints. While there is no known cure for arthritis, there are ways to manage the symptoms through lifestyle changes, including a healthy diet. The Arthritis Kitchen cookbook is designed to provide delicious and nutritious recipes that are specifically tailored to help manage arthritis symptoms.

This cookbook is not just about food; it is about living with arthritis and finding joy in the kitchen despite the challenges of the disease. Whether you are a seasoned cook or a beginner in the kitchen, this cookbook will guide you through easy-to-follow recipes that are both healthy and tasty. From breakfast to dinner, you will find a variety of recipes that will satisfy your cravings and support your health.

The Arthritis Kitchen is more than just a cookbook. It is a resource for those who want to take control of their arthritis symptoms through nutrition. By providing easy-to-understand information about the relationship between food and arthritis, this cookbook empowers readers to make informed decisions about their diet and lifestyle. It is a comprehensive guide to understanding the role of nutrition in managing arthritis symptoms, with practical tips and advice for incorporating healthy eating habits into daily life.

Through The Arthritis Kitchen, readers will discover how to enjoy delicious, healthy meals while managing their arthritis symptoms. With a variety of recipes that cater to different tastes and dietary restrictions, this cookbook will help readers create flavorful and satisfying meals that support their overall health and well-being.

Causes

Arthritis is a term used to describe inflammation and pain in the joints. There are many different types of arthritis, and the causes of each can vary. Some of the most common causes of arthritis include:

1. Age: As we age, the wear and tear on our joints can lead to arthritis. Over time, the cartilage in our joints may wear down, causing bones to rub together and leading to pain and inflammation.

2. Genetics: Some types of arthritis, such as rheumatoid arthritis, are believed to have a genetic component. This means that if you have a family history of the condition, you may be more likely to develop it.

Copyright © 2023 by Alice Caroline

All rights reserved. No part of this publication may be reproduced, distributed, or transmitted in any form or by any means, including photocopying, recording, or other electronic or mechanical methods, without the prior written permission of the publisher, except in the case of brief quotation embodied in critical reviews and certian other noncommercial uses permitted by copyright law.

Table of Contents

3. Injuries: Injuries to the joints can also lead to arthritis. This can include injuries from sports, accidents, or other trauma.

4. Infection: Certain infections can cause arthritis. For example, Lyme disease is known to cause joint pain and inflammation.

5. Autoimmune disorders: Some types of arthritis are caused by an overactive immune system. In these cases, the body attacks its own tissues, including the joints.

6. Lifestyle factors: Certain lifestyle factors, such as obesity and a lack of physical activity, can also contribute to the development of arthritis. Carrying excess weight puts extra strain on the joints, while physical activity helps to keep joints healthy and mobile.

It is important to note that the causes of arthritis can vary depending on the type of arthritis in question. For example, osteoarthritis is primarily caused by wear and tear on the joints, while rheumatoid arthritis is an autoimmune disorder.

In addition, there may be multiple factors at play when it comes to the development of arthritis. For example, a person may have a genetic predisposition to the condition, but lifestyle factors such as obesity or lack of physical activity may trigger its onset.

Understanding the causes of arthritis is an important step in managing the condition. By identifying the underlying causes, individuals may be able to make lifestyle changes or receive appropriate medical treatment to help manage their symptoms and slow the progression of the condition

Types of arthritis

The two most common types of arthritis are osteoarthritis and rheumatoid arthritis.

1. Osteoarthritis is a degenerative joint disease that results from wear and tear on the joints over time. It occurs when the cartilage that cushions the ends of bones in a joint begins to break down, causing bones to rub against each other. This can lead to pain, stiffness, and loss of mobility in the affected joint. Osteoarthritis most commonly affects weight-bearing joints like the knees, hips, and spine, but can also affect other joints like the hands and feet.

2. Rheumatoid arthritis, on the other hand, is an autoimmune disorder that occurs when the immune system mistakenly attacks the lining of the joints, causing inflammation. This inflammation can damage the cartilage and bone within the joint, leading to pain, swelling, and stiffness. Rheumatoid arthritis can also affect other parts of the body, such as the lungs, heart, and eyes. It typically affects the same joints on both sides of the body, such as the hands, wrists, and knees.

3. Other common types of arthritis include psoriatic arthritis, which is associated with the skin condition psoriasis; gout, which occurs when uric acid crystals build up in the joints; and lupus, an autoimmune disorder that can affect many different parts of the body, including the joints.

How Diet Affects Arthritis Symptoms

The foods that we eat can have a significant impact on our health, including our joint health. Certain foods can help to reduce inflammation and pain, while others can exacerbate arthritis symptoms. Here are some ways that diet can affect arthritis symptoms:

Inflammation

Inflammation is a key factor in the development and progression of arthritis. Certain foods can trigger inflammation in the body, leading to increased pain and stiffness in the joints. On the other hand, anti-inflammatory foods can help to reduce inflammation and ease arthritis symptoms.

Foods that can trigger inflammation include:

1. Processed and packaged foods that are high in sugar, salt, and unhealthy fats
2. Fried foods and fast food
3. Red meat and processed meats
4. Refined carbohydrates like white bread, pasta, and rice
5. Dairy products

Anti-inflammatory foods, on the other hand, include:

Fruits and vegetables, especially those that are rich in antioxidants like vitamin C and beta-carotene

Fatty fish like salmon, mackerel, and tuna, which are high in omega-3 fatty acids

Nuts and seeds

Whole grains like brown rice, quinoa, and whole wheat bread

Herbs and spices like ginger, turmeric, and garlic, which have natural anti-inflammatory properties

By focusing on a diet that is rich in anti-inflammatory foods and low in pro-inflammatory foods, people with arthritis may be able to reduce inflammation in their bodies and experience fewer symptoms.

Weight Management

Maintaining a healthy weight is important for people with arthritis because excess weight can put extra strain on the joints and exacerbate arthritis symptoms. Losing weight can help to reduce pain and improve mobility, but it can be challenging for people with arthritis to exercise regularly and follow a healthy diet.

One strategy for weight management is to focus on eating a balanced diet that is high in nutrient-dense foods like fruits and vegetables, whole grains, and lean protein. These foods can help to keep you feeling full and satisfied while providing your body with the nutrients it needs to function properly.

Another strategy is to be mindful of portion sizes and avoid overeating. Using a food scale or measuring cups can help you to keep track of your portions and ensure that you are not consuming more calories than you need.

Gut Health

The health of our gut microbiome – the community of bacteria that live in our digestive system – can also affect arthritis symptoms. Studies have shown that people with arthritis may have an imbalance in their gut bacteria, which can contribute to inflammation and other health issues.

To support gut health, it is important to eat a diet that is rich in fiber, which can help to promote the growth of healthy gut bacteria. Foods that are high in fiber include fruits and vegetables, whole grains, nuts and seeds, and legumes.

Probiotic foods, which contain live bacteria that can help to support gut health, can also be beneficial for people with arthritis. Examples of probiotic foods include yogurt, kefir, kimchi, sauerkraut, and kombucha.

Omega-3 Fatty Acids

Omega-3 fatty acids are a type of polyunsaturated fat that is essential for overall health. These fats have been shown to have anti-inflammatory properties, which can be beneficial for people with arthritis. Studies have found that consuming omega-3 fatty acids can help to reduce inflammation and pain in people with rheumatoid arthritis and other types of inflammatory arthritis.

Omega-3 fatty acids are found in fatty fish like salmon, mackerel, and tuna, as well as in walnuts, flaxseed, chia seeds, and other plant-based sources. For people with arthritis, it may be helpful to consume at least two servings of fatty fish per week or to take an omega-3 supplement.

Vitamin D

Vitamin D is important for bone health and may also have anti-inflammatory properties that can benefit people with arthritis. Studies have found that people with low levels of vitamin D are more likely to develop rheumatoid arthritis and other types of autoimmune diseases.

Vitamin D can be obtained from sunlight, fortified foods like milk and cereal, and supplements. For people with arthritis, it may be helpful to talk to a healthcare provider about whether vitamin D supplementation is necessary.

Calcium

Calcium is another nutrient that is important for bone health. People with arthritis may be at higher risk for osteoporosis, a condition that causes bone loss and increases the risk of fractures. Consuming adequate calcium can help to maintain bone density and reduce the risk of osteoporosis.

Calcium can be obtained from dairy products, leafy green vegetables, and fortified foods like cereal and orange juice. For people with arthritis, it may be helpful to consume at least 1,000-1,200 milligrams of calcium per day, depending on age and gender.

Vitamin C

Vitamin C is an antioxidant that is important for overall health and may also have anti-inflammatory properties. Studies have found that people with higher levels of vitamin C are less likely to develop rheumatoid arthritis and other types of inflammatory arthritis.

Vitamin C is found in fruits and vegetables, especially citrus fruits, strawberries, kiwi, and bell peppers. For people with arthritis, it may be helpful to consume at least 75-90 milligrams of vitamin C per day.

Magnesium

Magnesium is a mineral that is important for muscle and nerve function, as well as bone health. Studies have found that people with arthritis may be at higher risk for magnesium deficiency, which can contribute to muscle cramps, weakness, and other symptoms.

Magnesium is found in leafy green vegetables, nuts and seeds, whole grains, and beans. For people with arthritis, it may be helpful to consume at least 300-400 milligrams of magnesium per day.

Processed and Packaged Foods

Processed and packaged foods are often high in sugar, salt, and unhealthy fats, which can contribute to inflammation and exacerbate arthritis symptoms. These foods may also contain additives and preservatives that can be harmful to overall health. Instead, opt for whole, minimally processed foods like fruits, vegetables, whole grains, and lean protein.

Red and Processed Meats

Red and processed meats like beef, pork, and sausage contain high levels of saturated fat, which can contribute to inflammation and joint pain. These meats may also contain advanced glycation end products (AGEs), which are compounds that form when meat is cooked at high temperatures. AGEs have been shown to contribute to inflammation and may worsen arthritis symptoms.

Sugar-Sweetened Beverages

Sugar-sweetened beverages like soda and energy drinks are high in added sugar, which can contribute to inflammation and exacerbate arthritis symptoms. These beverages may also contain high-fructose corn syrup, which has been linked to increased inflammation and insulin resistance.

Fried Foods

Fried foods like french fries, fried chicken, and onion rings are often high in unhealthy fats and calories, which can contribute to inflammation and exacerbate arthritis symptoms. These foods may also contain advanced glycation end products (AGEs) that can contribute to inflammation and joint pain.

Alcohol

Alcohol can increase inflammation in the body and may worsen arthritis symptoms. Additionally, excessive alcohol consumption can increase the risk of osteoporosis, a condition that is more common in people with arthritis. While moderate alcohol consumption may not be harmful for everyone, it is important to talk to a healthcare provider about individual recommendations.

Gluten

Gluten is a protein found in wheat, barley, and rye. Some people with arthritis may have a sensitivity to gluten, which can contribute to inflammation and exacerbate arthritis symptoms. Additionally, some research suggests that following a gluten-free diet may help to reduce inflammation in people with rheumatoid arthritis.

Nightshade Vegetables

Nightshade vegetables like tomatoes, peppers, and eggplant contain a compound called solanine, which has been shown to aggravate inflammation in some people with arthritis. While not everyone with arthritis will have a negative response to nightshade vegetables, it may be helpful to limit or avoid these foods if they exacerbate symptoms

Banana Date Protein Muffins

Ingredients:

2 ½ cups old-fashioned oats

1 cup 1% plain Greek yogurt

2 eggs

½ cup sugar

2 ripe bananas

2 tsp baking powder

1 tsp vanilla

½ tsp baking soda

1 tsp cinnamon

3 tbsp chia seeds

6 Medjool dates (pitted and halved)

Instructions

Preheat oven to 400°F and lightly grease a 12-cup muffin tin with oil or line with paper liners.

In a food processor or high-powered blender, add rolled oats and blend into oat flour.

Place the rest of the ingredients, except chia seeds and Medjool dates, into the food processor or high-powered blender until everything is mixed together.

Fold the chia seeds into the batter.

Divide batter evenly into muffin tin.

Place ½ Medjool date on top of each muffin.

Bake for 18-20 minutes or until toothpick comes out clean.

Raspberry Clafoutis

Ingredients:

2 cups (500 mL) unsweetened frozen raspberries

1 1/2 cups (375 mL) liquid egg substitute

1 1/4 cups (300 mL) 2% milk

1 cup (250 mL) all-purpose flour

3/4 cup (175 mL) granulated sugar

3 tbsp (45 mL) melted non-hydrogenated margarine

1 tbsp (15 mL) vanilla extract

1/2 tsp (2 mL) salt

Icing sugar (optional)

Low fat vanilla yogurt (optional)

Instructions:

Preheat the oven to 350°F (180°C).

Scatter the raspberries in a greased, 11-inch (28 cm) shallow baking dish with fluted edges.

Combine the eggs, milk, flour, sugar, margarine, vanilla and salt in a blender. Blend, on medium speed, scraping the pitcher once, for 30 seconds or until smooth. (Or, combine all ingredients in a bowl and whisk until smooth.)

Pour the batter evenly over the raspberries.

Bake for 40 minutes or until set.

Dust with icing sugar (if using). Slice into wedges and serve warm with a dollop of yogurt (if using)

Sweet Potato Dip

Ingredients:

1 large sweet potato (about 1 lb/500 g)

2 green onions, trimmed

1/2 cup (125 ml) low fat sour cream

1/4 cup (50 ml) light mayonnaise

1/4 cup (50 ml) lightly packed fresh coriander leaves

2 tsp (10 ml) chipotle flavoured hot sauce (approx.)

1/4 tsp (1 ml) each ground cumin, salt and pepper

Instructions:

Pierce the sweet potato several times with a paring knife. Place in the microwave. Cook on HIGH heat, turning over halfway through, for 8 to 10 minutes or until very tender. Cool to room temperature. Peel away and discard the skin; transfer the flesh to the bowl of a food processor.

Cut each onion into 4 pieces. Add the onions, sour cream, mayonnaise, coriander, hot sauce, cumin, salt and pepper to the cooked sweet potato. Blend until smooth. (Add extra hot sauce as preferred to adjust spiciness to taste.)

Let stand for at least 15 minutes to develop the flavours. Store in an airtight container for up to 3 days. Serve with fresh-cut vegetables and baked tortilla or pita chips. Makes 2 cups (500 mL) dip.

Turmeric-Infused Beef and Barley Soup

Ingredients:

½ lb stewing beef, cubed

2 tablespoons extra virgin olive oil

1 medium onion, chopped

1 tablespoon minced garlic

2 medium tomatoes or ½ can diced tomatoes

1 stalk celery, chopped

1 tablespoon minced ginger

½ tablespoon turmeric

½ cup pearl barley, rinsed

6 cups low-sodium beef or vegetable broth

Salt and black pepper to taste

Cilantro for garnish

Instructions

In a large saucepan, heat the olive oil over medium-high heat. Add onions, garlic and celery and cook until transparent.

Add the beef and brown evenly.

Reduce the heat to medium. Add 1 cup of broth and scrape the bottom of the pot. Add the remaining broth, barley, tomatoes, ginger, turmeric, salt, pepper, and bring to a boil.

Reduce the heat and simmer, stirring the soup occasionally, until the barley is fully cooked and the meat is tender, about 60 to 90 minutes (longer cooking time makes for more tender meat).

Serve in deep bowls and garnish with cilantro leaves.

Cinnamon Power Waffles

Ingredients:

2 cups rolled oats

10 large eggs

2 cups cottage cheese

1 banana

1 tbsp baking powder

2 tsp cinnamon

Instructions

In a food processor or high-powered blender, add rolled oats and blend into oat flour.

Add the remaining ingredients to the food processor or blender. Blend until mixed well.

Use ¼ - ½ cup of batter at a time to make the waffles in your waffle maker.

Top waffles with your favourite toppings – nut butter, sliced banana, a drizzle of honey or maple syrup. You could even add vanilla Greek yogurt with berries.

Soothing Osteoarthritis Tea

Ingredients

1 Piece of Ginger (Approx. 3cm in Length)

1 Lemon

1 tspTurmeric (Level Tsp)

1 tsp Honey (or Agave Nectar)

A Pinch of Cayenne Pepper

A Pinch of Freshly Ground Pepper

Directions

Step One

Stick the kettle on and fill a large glass (or large mug) with hot water. Start by grating the piece of ginger into it, then add the turmeric, cayenne pepper and the freshly ground pepper. Stir well for 2-3 minutes.

Step Two

Next, mix 1 teaspoon of honey (or agave nectar) into your tea and let it steep until it reaches your preferred drinking temperature. Make sure to stir it every now and then!

Step Three

finally, squeeze the lemon into the tea and stir

Grapefruit brulee

Ingredients

1 grapefruit

1 tbsp coarse sugar, divided

Fresh berries, for garnish

Fresh mint leaves, for garnish

Directions

Prep the grapefruit: Cut it in half, and then slice the fruit into segments. (To help stabilize the fruit, cut a little bit of the skin off the bottom.)

Sprinkle coarse sugar on both halves of grapefruit. Using a kitchen torch, melt the sugar. You want the sugar to turn deep golden brown and form a crust on top of the fruit.

Garnish with fresh berries and mint leaves. Enjoy!

Green smoothie

Ingredients

Spinach (two handfuls)

1/2 cup of Parsley

1/4 cup of avocado

1 tbsp hemp seeds

1/2 tsp turmeric

1/3 cup rasberries

1 medium apple

Water and ice

Instructions

Blend everything together and enjoy!

GIN-SOAKED RAISINS

INGREDIENTS

1cup golden raisin (do not substitute for any other dried fruit or color of raisin)

1 -2cup gin (enough to just cover the raisins)

DIRECTIONS

Before you get started, make sure to read the label of your gin to check that it is made from or includes juniper berries. This is critical!

Put the raisins in a shallow glass container and pour enough gin into it to just cover the raisins.

Cover the container with cheesecloth and allow to stand until the raisins absorb the gin and the remaining liquid evaporates, about one week.

Each day, eat NINE of these "drunken" raisins.

I have read that it might take six weeks for this remedy to work, so be patient.

Teh Halia

Ingredients

3 sticks fresh turmeric or 1/8 ounce/4 g dried, peeled and chopped

One thumb-size piece fresh ginger root, peeled and grated

Few pinches black pepper

1 cup whole milk

1 teaspoon black tea leaves

Palm sugar (or maple syrup or brown sugar)

Directions

Combine the turmeric, ginger and black pepper in a mortar and pound with the pestle until you get a smooth paste.

Combine the paste with the milk, 1 cup water and the tea leaves in a saucepan and simmer over low heat until the liquid is reduced by half, 10 to 20 minutes. Strain. Sweeten with palm sugar to taste, and stir.

Before drinking, pour the teh between two containers, holding them the maximum width apart to aerate the tea as much as possible and produce froth on top. Despite not having too much of a medicinal effect on the remedy, this is more than just a flamboyant whim. Aerating the mix improves its flavor by making it easier for your tongue to perceive the chemicals that give the drink its unique taste.

Make the teh up as you need it, and drink at once. Take daily to help with arthritis, aches and pains in the joints, psoriasis, Crohn's disease and other inflammatory conditions. The paste will keep for up to 1 month in the refrigerator.

Strawberry Coconut Bread

Ingredients

1 cup Gluten Free All Purpose Flour blend (I used Robin Hood flour)

¼ cup coconut flour

½ cup granulated sugar

¼ cup icing sugar

1½ teaspoon gluten free baking powder

½ teaspoon baking soda

½ teaspoon salt

½ cup coconut yogurt

¼ cup Earth Balance (or any dairy free spread)

½ teaspoon pure vanilla extract

2 large eggs

½ cup strawberry, puree (may use fresh or frozen)

1 cup apples, puree

Instructions

Preheat oven to 350 F. Grease a bread loaf pan using a vegetable oil spray or PAM baking spray.

Remove the stems of the strawberries and cut them in half. You may also use frozen strawberries, especially in the winter time. Puree the strawberries in a food processor. My personal favourite is the NinjaMaster Pre Pro System.

Peel the apples using a vegetable peeler with a larger grip for your comfort. Cut the apple into quarters, cut out the core and puree them in food processor.

In a large bowl, cream vegetable spread and sugar together. Add the vanilla extract and mix until thoroughly combined. Add one egg at a time to the mixture until combined.

In a medium bowl add the gluten-free flour, baking powder, baking soda, salt.

Add the dry ingredients to the creamed vegetable spread mixture. Mix until fully combined

Add the strawberry puree, apple puree and coconut yogurt to the cake batter. Mix until fully combined.

Pour mixture into greased pan. Bake for 35-40 minutes. Check your bread because all ovens are different. Use a toothpick to check if the centre is done.

Cool completely before serving.

Beef bone broth

INGREDIENTS

2 lbs beef marrow bones, thawed, grassfed preferable

3 large carrots, unpeeled

1/2 medium celery root

a few sprigs of herbs – rosemary, oregano & thyme

2 bay leaves

2 tbsp apple cider vinegar, unpasteurized

1/2 tsp sea salt

water as needed

INSTRUCTIONS

Preheat oven to 425 degrees F

Place your bones onto a baking sheet and place into the oven. Cook for 30 minutes.

Wash and chop veggies into large pieces — large enough that they won't turn to mush.

Once your bones have roasted, pull them out of the oven and put them directly into a slow cooker. Add the veggies and the herbs into the cooker with the bones

Fill a 6-quart slow cooker with fresh water up to about ¾ inch under the rim. Add the bay leaves, ACV and salt

Cook in your pot on low. Remove the herbs after about 4 hours and remove the veggies once they're very soft, but not yet mushy

Let the bones cook for a total of 24-48 hours. Strain the broth, let cool a bit, and store in glass jars for up to ONE WEEK in your fridge. You can also freeze the broth if you don't use it right away.

Bone Broth Soup

Ingredients

1 medium onion, finely chopped

4 cups small, organic broccoli florets

1 cup cooked pearled barley

3 ½ cups homemade bone broth

2 garlic cloves, minced

2 tsp Italian seasoning

1 ½ cups water

1 tbsp olive oil

Salt and black pepper, to taste

Instructions

In a large pot heat the olive oil over medium heat.

Add the onion and cook for 5 minutes or until softened and translucent.

Add the broccoli, Italian seasoning, bone broth and water.

Bring the soup to a low boil.

Cover with a lid and cook until the broccoli florets are fork tender.

Add the cooked barley and cook for 1-2 minutes.

Remove from the heat.

Season with salt and black pepper to taste and serve

Dill & Mushroom Egg Cups

Ingredients

6 large eggs

⅔ cup homogenized milk or milk alternative

1 cup frozen vegetables

½ cup mushrooms, chopped

4 tbsp fresh dill, chopped

1 green onion stalk, chopped

½ cup cheddar cheese, grated or vegan alternative

black pepper, paprika and salt to taste

Instructions

Preheat oven at 350 degrees. Grease a 12-muffin tray with vegetable non-stick spray.

In a mixing bowl, whisk together the eggs, milk, paprika, salt and pepper. Add frozen vegetables, mushrooms, dill, green onions until thoroughly combined.

Pour the mixture into each of the muffin cups until each are filled.

Sprinkle each muffin cups with cheddar cheese.

Bake for 20 minutes.

Serve right away or store in airtight container for up to four days in the fridge or up to one month in the freezer.

Oatmeal

Ingredients

1 cup Gluten Free Oats

1 tbsp coconut oil

2 cups water

¼ tsp salt

1 tbsp cinnamon, powder

¼ tsp nutmeg, powder

1 tbsp flax seeds

1 cup quinoa, cooked

3 cups almond or soy milk (or any other milk alternative)

⅓ cup sweet potato, baked

¼ cup shredded coconut, unsweetened

1 tsp vanilla extract

¼ walnuts, chopped

2 tbsp Maple Syrup (optional)

Instructions

In a saucepan over medium heat, start by toasting the oat flakes on coconut oil until they are slightly brown.

Add water, salt, cinnamon and nutmeg. Bring to boil until oats are cooked.

Reduce heat to low and add almond milk, cooked quinoa, coconut, sweet potato, and vanilla extract. Bring to boil and let it simmer for five minutes.

Remove from heat and let stand covered for 5 minutes. Serve immediately, add extra almond milk, walnuts and maple syrup if desired.

Ginger Flax Quinoa Oatmeal

Add raisins or cranberries instead of sweet potato

Add ginger powder instead of cinnamon

Add 1 tsp of high quality Omega 3 oil. I use NutraSea as it doesn't have a strong fish after taste. Make sure you add it to the individual serving, not while cooking.

Crunchy Quinoa Oatmeal

Add Chia seeds instead of flax seeds

Sprinkle with roasted nuts or gluten free KIND honey clusters or gluten free granola for some crunch

Baked Avocado Egg

Equipment

Pizza Peel

Ingredients

2 avocados cut, halved with some of the centers spooned out. Large avocados work better, but whatever is accessible to you works just as well.

4 eggs

1-2 green onions, chopped

4 tbsp feta cheese, grated

Paprika, dried basil, salt and pepper to taste

2 tbsp Extra Virgen Olive Oil (EVOO)

Instructions

Fill each avocado half with an egg. It's easier to pour the eggs in a medium bowl and scoop out the egg yolks to put in the avocados.

Add green onions, paprika, salt, pepper, dried basil and drizzle with EVOO

Bake in a preheated oven at 425 °F for 15 to 20 mins, more or less based on your doneness preference.

Add feta cheese and serve immediately.

Fattoush Salad

Ingredients

4 slices of whole-grain gluten-free bread or gluten-free pita bread

4 radishes, thinly chopped (as arthritic humanly possible)

4 green onions, chopped

2 medium tomatoes, chopped

1 small cucumber, chopped or sliced

¼ cup feta cheese, crumbled (optional)

1 can light tuna in water (optional)

½ can chickpeas, drained and rinsed

½ medium green pepper, chopped

¼ cup finely chopped fresh parsley

⅓ cup finely chopped fresh mint or 2 teaspoons of dried mint

For Vinaigrette:

1-2 teaspoons minced garlic

salt and black pepper to taste

¼ cup fresh lemon juice

¼ cup of extra virgin olive oil

Instructions

Toast the bread, just enough to turn them golden and crisp, break into pieces. Set aside.

In a large salad bowl, combine the tomatoes, cucumber, green pepper, onions, chickpeas, tuna (if used), parsley, mint. Toss well.

In a small bowl, whisk together the ingredients for the vinaigrette, minced garlic, salt, pepper, lemon juice and olive oil.

Pour half of the vinaigrette to the tomato mixture and marinate for about 30 minutes in the fridge.

Fold in the toasted bread. Add the remaining vinaigrette and toss well. Top with feta cheese (if used). Serve immediately.

Parmesan Polenta and Eggplant

Ingredients

1 18-oz tube polenta

1 large eggplant

2 large eggs

¾ cup oat flour

1 tablespoon parsley, dried

1 tablespoon oregano, dried

1¼ cup parmesan cheese, grated

Instructions

Preheat oven at 425 °F and prepare a baking sheet with parchment paper. You may need two separate baking sheets.

Slice polenta into slices of ½ inch thick. It yields about 14 slices.

Slice eggplant into slices of ¼ inch thick.

In a shallow bowl, add the eggs and whisk or beat with a fork.

In a separate bowl, mix the oat flour, parmesan cheese, parsley and oregano.

Dip each polenta and eggplant slice in the egg. Cover all sides. Lift each slice up and let any excess egg drip off back into the bowl.

Coat each slice with the parmesan and oat flour mixture. Press the mixture into the top, bottom and sides of the slice.

Place the polenta slices on one baking sheet and the eggplant slices on the other baking sheet.

Bake for 20 minutes or until the polenta and eggplant appear crispy and golden.

Chickpea Salad

Ingredients

1-19 fl oz can chickpeas, low sodium, washed and rinsed

1 medium potato, peeled, cooked, diced

1 large tomato, diced

1 small onion, diced

½ cup cilantro, fresh, chopped

⅓ cup mint, fresh, chopped

⅓ cup tamarind or plum sauce

½ tablespoon fruit chaat masala seasoning (often includes mango powder, cumin, coriander, dried ginger, salt and black pepper) *see note below

Juice from ½ a lime

Sprinkle salt to taste (optional)

Instructions

In a medium bowl, mix together lime juice and tamarind (or plum) sauce.

Add in tomatoes, onions, cilantro, mint, and chaat masala spices. Combine all ingredients.

Mix in the chickpeas and cooked diced potatoes.

Serve at room temperature or chilled.

Souvlaki Paneer Kebabs

Ingredients

2 tablespoons extra virgin olive oil

¼ cup lime juice

¼ cup plain Greek yogurt

2 tablespoons soy sauce

¼ teaspoon salt

1 teaspoon pepper

1 tablespoon minced garlic

Kebabs

8 wooden skewers

1 piece of Paneer, about 12 oz, cut into bite-sized squares (approx. 28 cubes)

1 small red onion, quartered, segments separated

1 medium red pepper, cut into bite-sized pieces

14 cherry tomatoes

1 small zucchini, thickly sliced

Instructions

Soak wooden skewers in water for 30 minutes to avoid burning in the oven.

Preheat oven at 425 °F and prepare a baking sheet with aluminum foil.

Dressing: In a small bowl, whisk together olive oil, lime juice, yogurt, soy sauce, salt, pepper, and garlic. Set aside.

Kebabs: Arrange paneer and vegetables onto the skewers. Each skewer should have between 3 and 4 pieces of paneer alternating with assorted vegetables.

Place kebabs on the baking sheet and coat them generously with the dressing.

Roast for about 12-15 minutes or until cheese starts melting.

Cocoa Chia and Hemp Goodness

Ingredients

3 tablespoons Chia seeds

3 tablespoons Hemp Hearts

1 cup coconut milk (or your choice of plant-based beverage)

1-2 tablespoons cocoa nibs

½ teaspoon ground cinnamon

1 tablespoon shredded coconut (optional)

1 teaspoon maple syrup or honey (optional)

Fruit of choice

Instructions

Combine all ingredients in a bowl and stir with a whisk. Pour it into a mason jar and let it sit for two hours or overnight in the fridge. Add your favourite toppings.

Whole-Grain Breakfast

Ingredients

½ cup red quinoa, rinsed (I used Quinoa Royal by Go go Quinoa)

⅓ cup certified gluten-free rolled oats (Only Oats)

⅓ cup wild rice, rinsed

2 tablespoons Chia seeds

4 tablespoons Hemp Hearts

¼ cup raisins or dried cranberries

¼ cup chopped dried apricots

1 tablespoon cinnamon, powder

¼ teaspoon ginger, powder

¼ teaspoon salt

½ tablespoon Extra Virgin Olive Oil

2½ cups almond milk

1½ cups water

2 tablespoon maple syrup (optional)

Fruit of choice

Cashews (optional)

Instructions

Press the Sauté button and adjust time to 2 minutes; sauté chia and hemp seeds in olive oil.

Add quinoa, oats, rice, raisins, dried apricot, cinnamon, ginger, salt, almond milk, and water. Stir and mix all ingredients. Secure the lid and move pressure release valve to Sealing position

Press the Pressure Cook button at high pressure and adjust the time to 8 minutes.

When the timer beeps, use natural release. Remove bowl from pot. Mix well. Serve with additional almond milk, raisins, maple syrup and cashews if desired.

Maple Cornbread

Ingredients

¾ cup gluten-free whole-grain cornmeal flour (Bob's Red Mill)

1 cup all-purpose gluten-free flour (I used Robin Hood flour)

⅓ cup packed brown sugar

⅓ cup Canadian maple syrup

¾ teaspoon salt

3 teaspoons gluten-free baking powder

1 egg, room temperature

¼ cup Extra Virgin Olive Oil

⅓ cup plain yogurt (or cultured coconut yogurt)

¾ cup lactose-free milk (or your preferred plant-based beverage)

Instructions

Pre-heat oven to 400 F and grease an 8"x8" square baking pan.

Pre-heat oven to 400 F and grease an 8"x8" square baking pan.

Place the egg in a medium bowl. Use an electric mixer on low-medium speed until the egg turns a pale yellow. Add olive oil, sugar and maple syrup. Mix together until combined.

Add dry ingredients slowly into the mixture and mix until combined.

Add yogurt and milk at low speed until combined. Let the mixture sit in the fridge for 15 minutes.

Pour the batter into the greased pan. Bake for 20-25 minutes until a tester inserted into the middle of the bread comes out clean. Remove the cornbread from the heat and let it cool for 10-15 minutes before serving.

Infused Golden Milk

Ingredients

2 cups coconut milk (I used Silk coconut milk)

2 tablespoons pure maple syrup

2 teaspoons ground turmeric

½ teaspoon ground ginger

½ teaspoon cinnamon powder

½ teaspoon vanilla extract

½ teaspoon ground black pepper

2 mil CBD oil (currently using Redecan CBD Reign Drops 1:30)

Instructions

In a medium saucepan over medium heat, add all ingredients, except for the CBD oil.

Bring to boil; stir sparingly. Allow boiling for about one minute.

Turn the heat to low and allow the golden milk to simmer for 10 minutes.

After 10 minutes, turn off the heat and whisk in the CBD oil.

Enjoy immediately.

Spicy Shrimp

Ingredients

4 tablespoon Extra Virgen Olive Oil (EVOO)

3 Roma tomatoes, diced

½ medium onion, chopped

1 tablespoon garlic, chopped or garlic paste

2 tablespoons ginger, grated

1 Jalapeño pepper, chopped, seeded (optional)

1 teaspoon each coriander powder, turmeric powder, cumin powder, red pepper flakes

½ teaspoon chaat masala (optional)

Salt and pepper to taste

½ red bell pepper, chopped

½ green bell pepper, chopped

½ tablespoon lemon juice

16 ounces lemon juice

Chopped cilantro, cooked basmati rice or gluten-free tortilla

Instructions

Heat olive oil over a large saucepan over medium heat. Add onions and saute until translucent. Gently add the tomatoes. Stir the tomatoes and onions and let them cook for about 2 minutes.

Add garlic, ginger, coriander powder, turmeric, cumin, red pepper flakes and chat masala (optional). Simmer in low-medium heat for about 10 minutes. Stir the mix and add 1/4 cup of water if needed.

Add bell peppers and Jalapeno pepper (optional). Cook for 2 minutes. Add shrimp, coriander, and lemon juice. Mix well and cook for 5 minutes

Serve with basmati rice, wild rice or gluten-free corn tortilla.

Rice Pudding

Ingredients

4 cups Almond milk (or your favourite plant-based beverage), unsweetened

½ teaspoon vanilla extract

2 cinnamon sticks

1 cup parboiled rice, washed

¼ cup golden Sultana raisins

¼ cup shredded coconut, unsweetened

¼ cup raw cane sugar

1 teaspoon lemon zest

4 cloves (optional)

Instructions

In a large saucepan over medium heat, add almond milk and bring it to boil with the vanilla extract and cinnamon sticks.

Add rice, raisins, shredded coconut, raw cane sugar, cloves (optional) and lemon zest. Stir every 3 or 4 mins with a wooden spoon.

The rice pudding starts to thicken after 20-25 mins. You may add extra almond milk if it gets too thick and cook for 10 more minutes over medium-low heat.

Let it cool down for 5 mins. Serve hot. Sprinkle cinnamon powder and shredded coconut. You may also enjoy this rice pudding cold.

Chia Jam

Equipment

Small saucepan

Potato masher (optional)

Ingredients

½ cup frozen berries or berries about to go bad (washed)

2 tablespoons chia seeds

1 teaspoon vanilla extract

½ teaspoon cinnamon, powder

½ tablespoon pure maple syrup (optional)

1-2 teaspoon[s] Hemp Hearts (to sprinkle on toast)

Banana slices (optional)

Instructions

Heat a small saucepan over medium heat.

Pour berries into the pan and let them defrost, and release water.

Mash the berries with a fork or a potato masher (arthritis-friendly).

Turn heat down to low to prevent the berries from burning.

Once the berries are mashed, add chia seeds and mix them into the berries.

Allow the chia seeds to thicken up with the berry liquid.

Add in maple syrup, vanilla and cinnamon.

Mix thoroughly & enjoy!

Crispy Quinoa

Equipment

Baking tray

Mixing bowl

Serving bowls

Ingredients

1 cup quinoa, rinsed and drained

1 tbsp maple syrup or honey

1.5 tbsp hemp oil

1.5 tbsp plain Greek-style yogurt

1 cup mixed fresh seasonal fruit

4 tbsp crushed cashews, unsalted (optional)

Instructions

Preheat oven to 400°F. Mix quinoa with maple syrup and oil; spread in an even layer on a rimmed baking sheet. Bake until crisp for 13-15 minutes, stirring occasionally. Let it cool and transfer to a plate.

To serve, divide yogurt into two bowls, and top each with fruit, 4 tablespoons of crispy quinoa and crushed cashews.

Zucchini Salad Bowl

Equipment

Spiralizer (if available)

Small bowl

Large bowl

Cutting board

Arthritis-friendly knife (click here for helpful tips)

Ingredients

1 medium zucchini ends trimmed

½ medium lime, juiced

1 tbsp extra virgin olive oil

1 tbsp balsamic vinegar (optional)

Salt and black pepper to taste

½ Hass avocado, diced

⅓ cup frozen edamame cooked (as per package instructions)

3 stalks of green onions, chopped

⅓ cup sliced Kalamata olives

Fresh oregano, parsley, and basil to taste (optional)

Instructions

Using a spiralizer, cut the zucchini into thin spaghetti-like strands. Trim the strands into bite-size lengths, about 8-inches long and place them in a large bowl.

In a small bowl, whisk together lime juice, olive oil, balsamic vinegar, salt, and pepper.

Add diced avocado, olives, edamame, green onions, and herbs to the work bowl. Mix in the vinaigrette.

Sprinkle crumbled feta cheese to taste.

Serve immediately!

Spice Hot Chocolate

Equipment

Saucepan

Frother or whisk

Measuring spoons

Ingredients

2 cups plant-based beverage

1 tablespoon unsweetened cocoa powder, preferably organic

1 tablespoon dark chocolate chunks

1 tablespoon maple syrup (optional)

¼ teaspoon ground cinnamon

¼ teaspoon ground nutmeg

cloves powder 3 or ¼ teaspoon

2 pinches cayenne pepper or add to taste

Instructions

In a small saucepan, pour your favourite plant-based beverage (i.e. almond, cashew, hemp). Whisk in cocoa powder, dark chocolate & maple syrup

Cook over medium heat, stirring constantly.

Continue whisking until all ingredients have melted. Add in the spices. Mix well.

Keep stirring till the beverage is fragrant, you may also use a frother to mix.

Pour into a mug. Sprinkle cinnamon and cayenne pepper if desired.

Flaxseed crusted salmon

Ingredients:

4 tbsp soy sauce   substitute (such   as tamari sauce   or   liquid aminos)

1 ½ tbsp garlic paste

1 lemon, juiced

1 tbsp Dijon mustard

2 tbsp extra virgin olive oil

Salt and black pepper to taste

4 salmon fillets, about 4 oz each

Flaxseed crust

¼ cup quinoa flakes

¼ cup whole flaxseeds

1 tbsp parsley, dried

1 tbsp oregano, dried

Instructions

In a medium bowl, combine the soy sauce substitute, garlic paste, lemon juice, mustard, olive oil, salt and pepper. Place salmon in the bowl and coat well with the mix. Cover with plastic wrap and refrigerate for up to 1 hour.

In a shallow bowl, mix the quinoa flakes, flaxseeds, parsley and oregano.

Preheat oven to 425°F. Prepare a baking sheet with non-stick foil.

Transfer the salmon fillet to the dry mixture. Gently press the salmon on all sides over the crumbs, so it sticks well.

Arrange salmon fillets in the baking tray. Bake for about 12-15 minutes, or until the fish flakes easily with a fork.

If you want a crispier crust, switch the oven setting to broil "high" for 1-2 minutes to crisp the top slightly.

Serve with a Mediterranean salad and garnish with lemon wedges. Enjoy!

Red Potato & Dill Salad

Ingredients:

Salad

12 small red potatoes, skin on

¼ teaspoon salt

1/3 cup red onion, finely chopped

1/3 cup red or green bell pepper, chopped

1 stalk celery, chopped

3 tablespoons fresh dill, chopped

Dressing

½ cup olive oil-based mayonnaise

2 tablespoons Dijon mustard

Salt and pepper to taste

Instructions

Wash potatoes with a brush under warm running water.

Chop potatoes into bite-sized pieces, leaving the skin on.

Place potatoes in a microwave-safe bowl with ¼ cup of water and a pinch of salt. Microwave for 4 to 5 minutes or until a fork can easily be inserted into the potatoes. Drain well.

In a large bowl, combine onion, peppers, celery, dill, and potatoes.

In a medium bowl, whisk together all the dressing ingredients.

Gently combine the dressing with the potato mixture.

Garnish with additional chopped dill, if desired.

Raspberry Clafoutis

Ingredients:

2 cups (500 mL) unsweetened frozen raspberries

1 1/2 cups (375 mL) liquid egg substitute

1 1/4 cups (300 mL) 2% milk

1 cup (250 mL) all-purpose flour

3/4 cup (175 mL) granulated sugar

3 tbsp (45 mL) melted non-hydrogenated margarine

1 tbsp (15 mL) vanilla extract

1/2 tsp (2 mL) salt

Icing sugar (optional)

Low fat vanilla yogurt (optional)

Instructions:

Preheat the oven to 350°F (180°C).

Scatter the raspberries in a greased, 11-inch (28 cm) shallow baking dish with fluted edges.

Combine the eggs, milk, flour, sugar, margarine, vanilla and salt in a blender. Blend, on medium speed, scraping the pitcher once, for 30 seconds or until smooth. (Or, combine all ingredients in a bowl and whisk until smooth.)

Pour the batter evenly over the raspberries.

Bake for 40 minutes or until set.

Dust with icing sugar (if using). Slice into wedges and serve warm with a dollop of yogurt (if using).

Leek and Spinach Soup with mackerel

Ingredients:

6 cups (1.5 L) vegetable

98 percent fat-free chicken broth

2 cups (200 g) mushrooms, sliced

2 leeks, thinly sliced

1/2 teaspoon garlic, minced

Canola oil spray

6 ounces (168 g) mackerel fillets (or firm tofu, cubed)

1 tablespoon (9 g) seafood seasoning

2 cups (40 g) fresh spinach leaves

How to make:

Bring broth to a boil and add mushrooms, leeks, and garlic. Reduce heat and allow the soup to simmer 15 minutes.

Meanwhile, spray a frying pan with canola oil and place over medium-high

heat.

Sprinkle the fish fillets (or tofu) with the seafood seasoning, and sear in the pan 2 to 3 minutes on each side.

Remove from heat, add to the soup, and simmer an additional 5 minutes.

Two to 3 minutes prior to serving, add the fresh spinach leaves and allow to soften and wilt.

Buckwheat Noodles with Peanut Sauce

Ingredients:

1 packet buckwheat noodles

Peanut sauce

1/4 cup coriander leaves

1/4 cup chopped peanuts

6 scallions (spring onions- white and green part chopped)

1 teaspoon salt

1 tablespoon olive oil

How to make peanut sauce?

Ingredients:

1 cup lite coconut milk

¼ cup creamy peanut butter

¼ cup freshly squeezed lime juice

3 garlic cloves, minced

2 tablespoons low-sodium soy sauce, or gluten-free soy sauce

grated fresh ginger

How to make peanut sauce?

In a blender or food processor, process the coconut milk, peanut butter, lime

juice, garlic, soy sauce, and ginger until smooth. keep refrigerated in a tightly

sealed container for up to 5 days.

Cook the buckwheat noodles in water, olive oil and salt – drain the water once cooked.

In a large bowl, toss the buckwheat noodles with the peanut sauce to coat.

Garnish with the cilantro, peanuts, and scallions.

Manhattan-Style Salmon Chowder

Ingredients:

¼ cup extra-virgin olive oil

1 red bell pepper, chopped skinless salmon with pin bones removed, and chopped into ½ inch pieces

2 (28-ounce) cans crushed tomatoes, 1 drained and 1 undrained

6 cups no-salt-added chicken broth

2 cups diced (½ inch) sweet potatoes

1 teaspoon onion powder

½ teaspoon sea salt

¼ teaspoon freshly ground black pepper

How to make:

In a large pot, heat the olive over medium-high heat until it shimmers.

Add the red bell pepper and salmon. Cook the fish and bell pepper for about 5 minutes, stirring periodically, or until the fish is opaque.

Add the sweet potatoes, tomatoes, chicken broth, onion powder, salt, and pepper.

Turn down the heat to medium after bringing to a simmer. Cook for about 10 minutes, stirring occasionally, until the sweet potatoes are soft.

Turmeric-Infused Beef and Barley Soup

Ingredients:

½ lb stewing beef, cubed

2 tablespoons extra virgin olive oil

1 medium onion, chopped

1 tablespoon minced garlic

2 medium tomatoes or ½ can diced tomatoes

1 stalk celery, chopped

1 tablespoon minced ginger

½ tablespoon turmeric

½ cup pearl barley, rinsed

6 cups low-sodium beef or vegetable broth

Salt and black pepper to taste

Cilantro for garnish

Instructions

In a large saucepan, heat the olive oil over medium-high heat. Add onions, garlic and celery and cook until transparent.

Add the beef and brown evenly.

Reduce the heat to medium. Add 1 cup of broth and scrape the bottom of the pot. Add the remaining broth, barley, tomatoes, ginger, turmeric, salt, pepper, and bring to a boil.

Reduce the heat and simmer, stirring the soup occasionally, until the barley is fully cooked and the meat is tender, about 60 to 90 minutes (longer cooking time makes for more tender meat).

Serve in deep bowls and garnish with cilantro leaves.

Spiced Fruit Salad

Ingredients:

1 medium Honeydew melon, cubed

2 fresh mandarin oranges or clementines, peeled and segmented

1 cup red or green seedless grapes, halved

½ cup pomegranate seeds

½ cup blueberries

1 medium apple, cubed

1 medium guava, cubed (optional)

1.5 tablespoons fruit chaat masala seasoning (often includes mango powder, cumin, coriander, dried ginger, salt and black pepper – see note below)

Instructions

Wash the honeydew's skin with a scrub brush under running water to avoid contaminants entering the fruit when cutting through it.

Slice the honeydew melon in half and remove the seeds. Remove the rind and chop the melon into bite-sized pieces. If cutting honeydew is difficult, have someone else cut it for you or try pre-cut fruit from the store.

In a large bowl, combine the honeydew, clementines, grapes, pomegranate seeds, blueberries, apple and guava (if using).

Add in chaat masala seasoning. Combine all ingredients.

Serve chilled.

Red Potato & Dill Salad

Ingredients:

Salad

12 small red potatoes, skin on

¼ teaspoon salt

1/3 cup red onion, finely chopped

1/3 cup red or green bell pepper, chopped

1 stalk celery, chopped

3 tablespoons fresh dill, chopped

Dressing

½ cup olive oil-based mayonnaise

2 tablespoons Dijon mustard

Salt and pepper to taste

Instructions

Wash potatoes with a brush under warm running water.

Chop potatoes into bite-sized pieces, leaving the skin on.

Place potatoes in a microwave-safe bowl with ¼ cup of water and a pinch of salt. Microwave for 4 to 5 minutes or until a fork can easily be inserted into the potatoes. Drain well.

In a large bowl, combine onion, peppers, celery, dill, and potatoes.

In a medium bowl, whisk together all the dressing ingredients.

Gently combine the dressing with the potato mixture.

Garnish with additional chopped dill, if desired.

Thai Butternut Squash and Coconut Soup

Ingredients:

2 ½ lb butternut squash (1 medium squash)

1 medium sweet potato

2 tablespoons extra virgin olive oil

1 medium onion, chopped

1 tablespoon minced garlic

¼ cup Thai red curry paste

Salt and black pepper to taste

2 ½ cups low-sodium vegetable broth

1 can coconut milk or 1 cup organic coconut milk

Garnish (optional)

2 tablespoons unsalted peanuts

1 stalk green onions, chopped

2 tablespoons chopped fresh coriander or cilantro

1 tablespoon lime juice

Instructions

Preheat oven at 400 °F and line a baking sheet with aluminum foil.

Place the whole butternut squash and sweet potato on the baking sheet and bake for 30-40 minutes to enhance the flavours. Baking squash and sweet potato beforehand will make them easier to peel and chop. Set the baked vegetables aside and let them cool.

Once cooled, scoop the flesh out of the butternut squash. Peel the sweet potato and cut in cubes.

In a large saucepan, heat the olive oil over medium-high heat. Add onions and cook until softened.

Add the baked squash and cubed potato to the saucepan. Cook for about five minutes, stirring occasionally.

Add the garlic and curry paste, stirring gently until the vegetables are well coated. Add the broth, cover and bring it to a boil.

Reduce heat to low and simmer for about 25 minutes, stirring occasionally. Remove from heat and let stand for 5 minutes.

Blend soup until smooth using a hand blender. Return the soup to medium heat and stir in the coconut milk. Add salt and black pepper to taste.

While soup cooks, combine peanuts, coriander, green onions, and lime juice in a small bowl (optional).

Ladle soup into deep bowls and garnish with peanut mixture (if using).

Conclusions

The Arthritis Kitchen offers a range of delicious and nutritious recipes that can help manage the symptoms of arthritis. By incorporating anti-inflammatory foods and nutrients into your diet, you can help reduce inflammation, ease pain and stiffness, and improve overall joint health.

Some key takeaways from the book include the importance of consuming omega-3 fatty acids, antioxidants, and fiber-rich foods, as well as avoiding or limiting processed foods, sugar, and saturated fats. The recipes are designed to be easy to prepare and enjoyable for everyone, whether you have arthritis or not.

In addition to the recipes, the book also provides valuable information on the science behind arthritis and how diet and nutrition can impact the disease. It is important to consult with a healthcare professional before making significant changes to your diet or lifestyle, especially if you have any underlying health conditions.

Overall, The Arthritis Kitchen is a valuable resource for anyone looking to improve their joint health and manage arthritis symptoms through a healthy and delicious diet.

www.ingramcontent.com/pod-product-compliance
Lightning Source LLC
Chambersburg PA
CBHW070756220526
45467CB00014B/610